Dr Graham Cure studied microbiology and biochemistry at the University of Reading and was awarded a PhD, in 1974. Subsequently, he worked in various scientific and technical positions in the food industry for over 40 years. He became interested in nutrition when advice from nutritionists failed to reduce his high blood cholesterol. Realising that there must be something wrong with the "science," he set about uncovering and correcting much of the misinformation that we see reported almost every day in newspapers and on television. Now over 70, he enjoys walking and tennis, and is faster around the tennis court than many people half his age.

To Margaret, William, Ailish, Alexandra and Lily

Dr Graham Cure

PROPER NUTRITION PROPERLY EXPLAINED

AUSTIN MACAULEY PUBLISHERS™

LONDON • CAMBRIDGE • NEW YORK • SHARJAH

A CIP catalogue record for this title is available from the British Library.

ISBN 9781398433267 (Paperback)
ISBN 9781398422568 (ePub e-book)

www.austinmacauley.com

First Published 2022
Austin Macauley Publishers Ltd®
1 Canada Square
Canary Wharf
London
E14 5AA

Table of Contents

Preface

Knowledge might be power, but understanding is better

Because I love eating, I often eat over 5000 Calories a day, yet I have a 32-inch (80 cm) waistline and a body mass index (BMI) of 22. I am 70 years old, yet I am faster around the tennis court than many people half my age. And I can walk faster than almost anybody. No, I am not an exercise fanatic; I have never run a marathon; in fact, I don't jog at all, and I've never been to a gym. Quite simply, I understand how the body deals with the energy we feed it and how to stop it from ending up as unsightly fat.

I am not impressed by most of the nutritional information disseminated by governments and nutritionists over recent decades. We had been told for over forty years that saturated animal fats cause heart disease, but suddenly and without explanation, we have recently been informed that it's the sugar that's the problem. We were told for decades not to eat more than three eggs a week as they contain a lot of cholesterol, and cholesterol causes heart disease, yet this advice suddenly disappeared as well. We have also been advised to eat a Mediterranean-style diet containing polyunsaturated oils. People who live near the Mediterranean consume mostly olive oil, which is predominantly a monounsaturated oil.

I am sure that, individually, nutritionists do the best they can with the tools with which they were provided during their training. The trouble is that the teachers' mistakes are passed down to the pupils, and that has mostly continued since modern nutrition became an accepted science some half a century ago. While nutrition courses teach students about carbohydrates, fats, and proteins, they rarely teach about how these nutrients are broken down, absorbed, and integrated into the body and hardly ever about how they interact with one another.

There are many problems with nutrition research today.

Firstly much of it is done or sponsored by an organisation with a vested interest. So fat companies sponsor research on fats, sugar companies sponsor research on sugar, and so on. I had some involvement with a sugar company back in the mid-1990s. They sponsored a piece of research done by a local university specifically to prove that sugar did not cause obesity. It was very easy for university researchers to "prove" that this was indeed the case!

Secondly, research is often done on a small number of people for cost reasons, and it is done over short timescales because everybody wants answers immediately. As a facetious example, this is the sort of thing that happens. The Jango Berry Marketing Company believes its berries are effective against FuFu disease, so it engages a university (and all universities are short of money) to do a quick bit of research. A few people with FuFu disease, often as few as twenty, are recruited and divided into two groups. One group is fed Jango berries for a few weeks, and the other group is fed a placebo. During the trial, the progress of the disease is monitored, and in the end, the researchers use statistics to determine whether there has been any improvement in the disease in the group fed Jango berries relative to the group fed the placebo. We have all heard of lies, dammed lies, and statistics, so the researchers manage to find a benefit (often a very minor one), and the results are published to tell us how good Jango berries are against FuFu disease, often with a headline in tomorrow's paper: "Jango berries cure FuFu disease." Yes, this may be slightly cynical, even possibly slightly exaggerated, but it's not a million miles from the truth.

Thirdly researchers using these statistical techniques often attempt to remove the distorting effects of "confounders." As the name suggests, these are other aspects of people's lifestyles that the researchers think might confuse the results, such as income, smoking, level of exercise, or obesity level. Picking different confounders to include or exclude from the statistics can change the results. According to a recently published study, the effect of taking a vitamin E supplement could apparently reduce death rates, have no effect, or increase death rates depending on which confounders were included or excluded from the statistics (1). At different times, other researchers have found similar discrepancies in the effect of vitamin E on prostate (2,3) and other cancers (4).

Fourthly there is something academics call "publication bias." Work that shows a significant result is more likely to be published than studies that show no effect. So a paper that shows a link between vitamin E intake and death rates is much more likely to be published than a paper that shows no link.

Thus scientists are driven to find a significant result even where one doesn't really exist. Researchers must stop such poor research; it may be good for their careers as they get more publications, but it is not good science. And the more publications a researcher has to their name, the more likely they are to get a better job.

Of course, there have been some excellent studies done over many years, sometimes over decades, and involving thousands of people, and those are the studies from which valid conclusions can certainly be drawn. But nobody wants to change their eating habits for years, so they are based on asking volunteers to keep food diaries and monitoring the volunteers' health over many years. This is not a recipe for timely results.

We need to find another way. Fortunately, I believe there is one. Researchers could analyse the "Jango" berry components, find out how these components interact in the body, and how they might affect the disease's progress. But this takes much longer, requires far more equipment, and dare I say a rather higher level of knowledge and expertise. We should strive to understand how all the dietary components interact with our body's workings and how a good diet can positively impact our overall physical and mental health rather than on just one specific disease.

Let's also remember that a well-balanced diet consists of scores of different foodstuffs that all interact in how the body deals with them. This is impossible to research just by looking at one component of the diet in isolation. The best way to do this is by looking inside the body at how all the various chemicals in our food are dealt with and interact, and this is a part of what biochemistry attempts to do.

I studied biochemistry. It is a long word and frightens many people, but it shouldn't as it's merely the study of the substances and processes that occur within living organisms, including man. This includes the processes involved in digesting and absorbing the components of the food we eat and, more critically, what happens to them once they enter our bloodstream and our body. Therefore, it seems strange that many nutrition courses, even today at degree level, contain little or in some cases no biochemistry at all. They concentrate instead on healthy eating guidelines, weight loss, fad diets, understanding food labelling, nutritional claims, sports and dietetic nutrition, food pyramids and energy optimisation. In fact, almost everything except what happens to the food when it enters our bloodstream.

As a biochemist, I fail to understand how anyone without extensive knowledge and particularly an understanding of biochemistry can consider themselves a nutrition expert. I am sure that if more biochemists had been more involved in the nutritional information disseminated over the last fifty years or so, many of the past misconceptions and mistakes would not have been made.

I also have some forty years' experience in the food industry. Since I started looking at nutrition through a biochemist's eyes, I have realised that many of the mantras we have been asked to accept as gospel simply must be wrong. So indeed must much of the information that we read in newspapers and magazines and hear on the television and even from governments. Much of it truly is "fake news". I find it unbelievable that many people will spend good money on a book on nutrition or healthy living just because a so-called celebrity writes it. While such people are undoubtedly masters of their own craft, what do they know or understand about nutrition? The fact that so many people have given their names to diets of one sort or another in recent years, many of which purport to make you thin in just a few weeks with very little effort, should surely set alarm bells ringing.

I am going to present nutrition through the eyes of a biochemist. I will try not to use long words or difficult concepts. Instead, I will try to lead us in simple and easy-to-understand everyday terms to explain what happens to the food we eat. In doing so, I apologise to any biochemists who might read this for its over-simplicity in that regard. One of the advantages of being seventy years old is that one is able to combine academic knowledge with intuition; one develops an instinct for what is likely to be right and what may not be; to sort the good from the indifferent.

Therefore, I aim to help the non-biochemist reader *understand* what I believe to be right. It is the understanding that is important rather than just the knowledge. We cannot go on just picking up sound bites every day or two from television, newspapers, or magazines without understanding how all of these parts fit together. I will not be prescriptive and say that you must eat this or must not eat that. Instead, I hope to give you the knowledge and understanding to help you make your own food choices.

This contrasts with what we read in newspapers, where today we are told that we should be eating this to ward off cancer. Tomorrow we are told that we should be eating something else for dementia, and the day after, it is yet something different for heart disease. Nobody takes the trouble to try to explain how it all fits together.

How to use this book

This is deliberately a small book, only some ninety pages long. I have tried not to use unnecessary words or to ramble. It won't take you long to read it, so I really do suggest that you read it slowly, making sure you absorb and understand it as you go. You might also consider re-reading it two or three times or, indeed, returning to it every few months to cement the knowledge and understanding in your own head. I cannot emphasise enough that it is the understanding of everything put together that will help you make good food choices and perhaps prolong your life and its quality in later years. Unfortunately, understanding means that the reader has to devote some quality time to reading and understanding, but surely this is worth it to improve the quality of your life and maybe to extend it.

But if you really are one of those people who don't care about the detail but just want to know what to eat, then, if you have to, skip to the final chapter, Putting It All Together, which summarises the information in the preceding chapters. However, I don't advise this as you will not get the understanding that is so important.

Remember also that there is no such thing as good or bad food, only a good or bad diet. You don't have to eat good stuff all the time; treats are permitted. I am certain that if everybody in the country were to understand nutrition and follow the simple guidelines given here, there would, after a couple of decades or so, be much less obesity, people would be much healthier and, in many cases, live longer. In time, the health service would save huge amounts of taxpayers' (that is your) money.

As this improvement in the nation's health will take at least a generation, we need to start with young children. We all know that childhood obesity has become a significant problem in recent years. It has occurred for two main reasons. Firstly it is because of poor nutrition, for which there is a tendency to blame the media, food companies, supermarkets, and governments, in fact, everybody but the parents themselves. Secondly, it is because of a sedentary lifestyle in many of today's youngsters. In part, this is because some people try to ban normal childhood activities such as running in playgrounds on rather silly health and safety grounds, and in part because of the long periods of time that many children (and adults) spend on electronic gadgets or watching television. At the very least, children should walk or cycle to and from school or enjoy an hour or so of playing outside each day. A good diet, a regime of exercise, and instilling in their children the reasons why these are necessary and enjoyable is perhaps the best education that parents can give their offspring. So parents and teachers need understanding.

Please note. This book is about nutrition and lifestyle, and I hope that the information may prolong your life and improve its quality. It is not intended to treat any medical issues you may have, for which you should see a qualified medical professional.

Much of the technical material presented here can be found in most standard biochemistry or medical textbooks. Although this is not intended to be an academic book, I have included a small number of some of the better recent scientific references and reviews at the end of the book. These are cross-referenced in the text by the numbers (1), (2) etc.

Energy

Don't bother counting Calories

Why do we eat?

We eat to produce energy. Energy is the ability of the body to perform work. As well as fuelling our everyday lives, energy is used to keep our heart, lungs, kidneys, liver, brain, and other vital organs working and keep our body temperature at about 37C (98.5F). So it follows that other things being equal, we generally need more energy for heat in winter than in summer and more energy if we keep our house and work environment cool. However, in summer, we may, of course, be outside enjoying fine weather and getting more exercise.

The energy available in food is measured in Calories.

What is a Calorie?

Many of us may remember from our school science that a calorie is a heat unit, specifically the heat required to raise one gram of water by one degree centigrade. This is not much, and so in nutrition, we use the Calorie (capital C), which is one thousand calories. The Greek for one thousand is kilo, so the correct term is kilocalorie or kcal as used in food labelling. A kilojoule (kJ) also found on food labels is 4.2 Calories.

So why is it that two people of similar ages and living similar lives can eat the same number of Calories, and one of them be slim and trim and the other overweight or even obese? Energy cannot simply disappear – that is a basic law of science – and so there can only be three possible reasons which we will examine in more detail as we move through:

1. Because the slim person *absorbs* fewer Calories into their body through the intestinal wall than the overweight person, even though they both eat similar numbers of Calories.
2. Because the slim person's body *deals* with the Calories they absorb more efficiently than the overweight person. We say that the slim person has a *faster metabolism*; that is, they produce more heat, which is why many people feel hot after a heavy meal.
3. Because the slim person *uses* more Calories, in other words, they do more exercise. This need not be highly active; it could be passive exercises such as housework or gardening.

From a biological standpoint, we should understand that the food in our gut is not yet part of our bodies. Our gut is simply a tube, albeit a highly sophisticated tube comprising mouth, throat, stomach, small and large intestines, and rectum, that runs through our body. In the middle of this tube is a non-sterile environment containing unabsorbed food and trillions of bacteria. It is a convenient way of carrying around our food. At the same time, we digest it, rather than living like a housefly that has to secrete digestive enzymes onto food outside its body and then wait until it has been partly digested before it can be sucked up. Food does not properly become part of our bodies until we absorb it; that is, it (minus the bacteria) passes across the tube boundary and into our body proper, which is normally sterile.

We all absorb calories at different rates and to a different extent for a lot of different reasons.

1 Because of short or long intestinal transit times,
2 The physical condition of our gut linings,
3 The amount and types of dietary fat we eat,
4 Differences in gut microflora (bacteria and yeasts),
5 The fibre content of the meal,
6 The sugar content of the meal,
7 The types of carbohydrate contained in the meal,
8 Whether we graze or eat large meals,
9 The water content of the meal and the water available in the gut,
10 Interaction of all the above.

The absorption of some nutrients can vary from as low as 10% of the amount ingested in some people to as much as 90% in other people (typically 50–80%), so there is little point in comparing calorie intake from one person to another, or indeed in counting the calories we eat at all. The only thing that matters is the number of calories we absorb (5).

As I said in the Preface, because I love eating, I regularly consume far more than I should, often around 5000 Calories a day, over twice the recommended amount for an adult male. I should, according to the Calorie counting theory, look like the side of a house. Yet I don't; I am a slim five feet ten inches

(178cm) with a 32-inch (81cm) waistline. Yes, I get a reasonable amount of exercise but not an excessive amount. Yes, I have good temperature control and normally feel warm, but without obviously sweating. So I have a reasonable but not excessively fast rate of metabolism. I am slim simply because I absorb only the Calories I need.

Calories that are absorbed are used to generate energy in our bodies. This energy comes from the three food groups: proteins, carbohydrates, and fats, as shown in Figure 1.

There are other important nutrients, including water, vitamins, minerals, and antioxidants, but these are not used to produce energy.

Carbohydrates

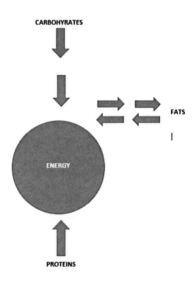

Figure 1. Energy is generated from carbohydrates and fats and sometimes from proteins

What are proteins?

Proteins are the building blocks of tissue and are used to grow and replace body tissues. Our bodies are constantly being renewed. Even something as solid as bone is completely replaced every seven to ten years, so today's bones have been completely renewed since about 2010. Proteins are used to replace the soft tissues in our bodies in much the same manner, sometimes very frequently. It is the way that nature has of keeping our bodies looking and feeling young.

Many older people might look at their wrinkled faces or twisted torsos and think that is not so. But consider that the human body works every second of every day from conception until the day we die, and if we look after ourselves, it can last for a hundred years or more. Even our best motor cars working for perhaps only an hour or two a day, on average last only ten or fifteen years.

So proteins are used for constant tissue renewal. Unless we have starved ourselves very severely for several days, not much protein is generally broken down to produce energy. Proteins can act as a fuel store but only at the expense of some muscle wastage.

So our energy comes mainly from the carbohydrates and fats we consume, as shown above, and as we discuss in the next chapter. Obviously, if we eat less fat, then unless we are prepared to go hungry, we will consume more carbohydrate and vice-versa to maintain our energy needs and feel replete. As we've been told for decades not to eat much fat, we must all be eating more carbohydrates than we did in the past. So let's look in more detail at the relationship between carbohydrates and fats.

Carbohydrates vs Fats

Don't worry about fat; it's the sugar that's the problem

Carbohydrates comprise the following:

Sugars such as glucose, sucrose (table sugar), fructose (fruit sugar), and lactose (milk sugar). There are also some other less well-known sugars,

Refined starches (which are generally white) such as white flour (used in bread, cakes, biscuits, and pasta), white rice and similar refined grains and potatoes and similar root vegetables without their skins,

Unrefined starches (which are generally brown) which include all of the above but with their husks or skins,

Soluble fibre which, as the name suggests, attracts water and which is usually reasonably soft, such as fibre in fruits, and

Insoluble fibre, which is usually quite hard such as that found in vegetables that generally need to be cooked to soften them.

Our bodies digest soluble fibre only quite poorly and insoluble fibre hardly at all. They become roughage. The transition between digestible carbohydrate and fibre is not very distinct. Think of the tiniest bit of sugar that can exist (scientists call it a molecule) as a bead. By analogy, a simple starch is a short string of beads (sometimes only two), as on a necklace or bracelet. The body breaks down these simple starches by cutting off the end bead, then the next and so on along the chain until all the carbohydrate is broken down to sugar.

However, as carbohydrates become more complex, the number of beads and the necklace length increases. Branching and cross-linking also occur so the threads can become woven or tangled. These long chains and sheets can then become folded into tight balls, and the body's enzymes that easily break down simpler carbohydrates physically cannot get in to find the ends and start breaking them down. It's a bit like trying the find the end of a ball of string, and if the body's enzymes can't find the end, the fibre remains undigested roughage.

Herbivorous animals that eat these complex plant fibres have developed specialised ways of dealing with them. For example, ruminants such as cows have four stomachs filled with highly specialised bacteria, that eventually extract some energy from this otherwise indigestible material. Rabbits have a huge appendix, also filled with specialised bacteria. Cows and sheep eat for many hours every day just to take in sufficient food to keep them alive, as the amount of energy extracted from grass is so small. We humans do not have these specialisms and simply cannot break down such fibre.

Fibre is, of course, very good for us. It provides our intestines with something to work on physically and keeps our lower gut healthy. It also "hides" Calories in its midst and prevents them from being absorbed so that relatively fewer Calories are absorbed from a high fibre diet than from a low fibre one. Without sufficient fibre, not only do we absorb more Calories but we also run the risk of becoming constipated and of not optimising our gut bacteria.

Let's turn to fats, but for the time being, forget long words like polyunsaturates and monounsaturates that some media people like to use to make themselves appear knowledgeable; I suspect that if you asked many of these people what these words actually mean, they probably wouldn't be able to tell you. It's much easier to think of the fats in our diet as coming from three sources: animal fats, plant oils, or fish oils. As the name suggests, animal fats are solid at room and, more importantly, at body temperature, much as they appear in beef, lamb, or pork in a butcher's shop. We have all seen the thick layers of fat on the outside of a lamb or pork loin chop, and in our own bodies, similar layers are deposited under the skin to help keep us warm, or elsewhere in the body, such as on the thighs or abdomen (white fat, used as an energy store). In more severe cases, fat can be deposited around organs such as the liver (visceral fat), which can be dangerous to health. As many of us know, once deposited, these fat layers are very difficult to remove. Brown fat is found in the neck and shoulder region and is used to create heat if we get cold.

In contrast, plant and fish oils, which are essential for good health, are obviously liquid at body temperature and are not stored as lumps of unsightly fat but are tucked out of sight and distributed throughout the body tissues. All chefs and housewives know that if you want to make a piece of meat really tender and succulent, you marinate it for an hour or two in olive or rapeseed oil before cooking. Not surprisingly, therefore, research has shown that an increase in the amount of plant oils increases the flexibility and softness of the cell membranes in our bodies and therefore in our tissues so that when we joke about our tired, aching bodies needing an oil, there just might be more than a grain of truth there. Yet for the past half a century or so, we have been urged to eat a low-fat diet.

Let's now look at two different meals to see how our bodies deal with a carbohydrate meal and a fat meal.

Breakfast

A large glass of fruit juice. From a nutritional standpoint, it doesn't matter if this is freshly squeezed, which obviously tastes better, or is from a packet of unsweetened juice. Bear in mind that fruits contain large amounts of sugar, and we'll return to this later.

Breakfast cereal. If you look at the packet, you will probably see that the first ingredient is wheat, and the second is sugar. Just for good measure, many of us sprinkle more sugar on top.

A slice or two of white toast, without butter as we've been told this is bad for us, so we smother it with jam or marmalade instead.

A couple of cups of tea or coffee with two or three spoons of sugar or a fizzy drink also containing lots of sugar.

As you've gathered, there's a lot of sugar here: around 20g even in a small glass of unsweetened juice, several spoons full in cereal, perhaps another 10g in jam or marmalade, and yet another 7–8g with every teaspoon of sugar in the tea or coffee. I know many people will be thinking that the fruit juice is fruit sugar (fructose), but in most common fruits such as apples and oranges, only about half the sugar is fructose, and the rest is other common sugars such as glucose and sucrose (table sugar). And once the fruit is squeezed and the fruit fibre left behind, these sugars, as we've seen, are absorbed by the body very quickly; indeed we can measure an increase in blood sugar fewer than fifteen minutes after ingestion.

All this sugar causes our blood glucose to rise. If this were to continue unchecked, we could go into a hyperglycaemic coma as do type 1 diabetics if they forgot to take their insulin. If we go immediately after breakfast for a long walk or cycle to school or work, for example, or run or swim or play some energetic sport, this glucose is converted into energy, and blood glucose returns to normal levels. Unfortunately, after breakfast, many of us sit in a chair, read the paper, watch breakfast television, get in the car, drive to work, or drive the children or grandchildren to school. Our blood glucose levels, therefore, continue increasing. Healthy individuals produce their own insulin in the pancreas, and that reduces blood glucose to normal levels.

But how does insulin do this? Our bodies don't store much carbohydrate. A small amount is stored in the leg muscles (about 350g or 3/4lb) and the liver (about 100g or 1/4lb) as a carbohydrate called glycogen that can be used by the body to produce instant energy if required (historically to escape predators, for example, or if our blood sugar is low). But today, in well-fed individuals, these glycogen stores are normally full except after heavy exercise, and if we just continue to sit in a nice warm house or car, we are not using many Calories.

So the body does the only thing it can do. Insulin works by turning on the chemistry that converts sugars into fats. Take another look at Figure 1 on page 18 and you'll see how this happens – the sugar and carbohydrate simply have nowhere else to go. And because biologically we are animals, it's turned into animal fat. Many people just don't realise that *most of the animal fat in our bodies is there because we make it, not because we eat it.* Indeed, if we significantly reduce the fat in our diets, we have to replace it with something or feel hungry. Protein is expensive, so normally the replacement food is carbohydrate. Even if there is not too much free sugar in the carbohydrate, the body will break the bead necklace down to sugar, and the end result will be stored animal fat. Quite clearly, there is a direct link between the significant decrease in fat intake and the consequent increase in carbohydrate intake over the past several decades and the increase in population obesity.

Because sugars are absorbed so quickly, within a few minutes of ingestion, we often feel hungry again very quickly. We settle down to coffee at about 11 o'clock and eat a scone or pastry with it, and the whole process starts all over again. Yet more animal fat gets deposited.

So suppose for lunch we have a very different sort of meal, one which contains a lot of fat, but with roughly equal quantities of animal fat, plant and fish oils. With the exception of the butter, many of us might now accept that this might be quite a healthy meal.

Lunch

In contrast to breakfast, we'll have a fatty meal.

A very thin slice of wholemeal bread (unrefined carbohydrate) containing lots of seeds, grains, and nuts on which we spread a thick layer of butter (not a spread as butter contains animal fat).

We'll add some lightly poached wild salmon, which contains some 10–15% fish oil (the rest is protein and water). Or smoked salmon, if you prefer.

We'll top it with plenty of avocado, which contains about 20% plant oil (the rest is mostly water and fibre).

There is very little carbohydrate in this meal, as there is no carbohydrate at all in fish (or meat for that matter). Because fats aren't soluble in water, they are absorbed much more slowly than sugars and carbohydrates; sugar and carbohydrate absorption is measured in a few minutes while fat absorption takes many hours.

Again chefs and housewives know that if you are making a pie with a pastry base and you want to stop the base going soggy, you rub a thin layer of butter or margarine over the pastry. This significantly slows the migration of moisture from the filling, whether it's meat or fruit, and the base remains drier for longer. Oils and soft fats like butter or margarine have a similar effect in our intestines, and they act as a barrier that significantly slows down the absorption of all foodstuffs. If you eat low fat diets, you lack much of a barrier layer and will almost certainly absorb many more Calories. You are likely to be heavier than if you eat a balanced diet containing a reasonable amount of fat and oils.

As we have said, sugars are absorbed in a few minutes while fats take hours, which is why fats are much more filling. That is why eating sugar when mixed with fat such as in chocolate or ice-cream raises blood sugar more slowly, typically one to two hours after eating. Eating the same quantity of sugar on its own or drinking a sugary drink or fruit juice causes a much quicker and higher peak in blood glucose levels only minutes after consumption.

Our extremely clever bodies realise that they need plant and fish oils as they cannot make them, so the body stores them for later use. They are known as essential fatty acids (EFAs) and their role will be explained in Chapter 7. So after a mixed fat meal, the body preferentially uses the animal fats in the butter to give it energy rather than the plant or fish oil. Because the butter is absorbed over a long period, the Calories are not suddenly rushed into the body but are released slowly over several hours as the body needs energy, so that little if any of the animal fat in the butter will be stored.

So perversely, a diet high in sugars and carbohydrates often results in deposits of animal fat, whereas a diet high in varied fats may not. Remember that *if you don't eat fat, you will inevitably eat more carbohydrates and will most likely put on more weight and start down the road to obesity.* Although many people find it difficult to believe this, if you eat only fat and protein and eliminate carbohydrate from your diet, you are almost certain to lose weight (by a process known as ketosis). This is the principle of the Atkins' diet. Fat by itself is not fattening.

I am not advocating any dieting, nor am I suggesting that you don't eat carbohydrates. My aim is to help you to understand what happens when you eat these different foodstuffs. I am suggesting that you take the time to understand what is happening when you eat and thus make informed food choices to eat a properly balanced diet. This is responsible nutrition advice.

So calls for a fat tax made a few years ago by many people who should have known better were unnecessary and indeed would have been unworkable. There is already a tax on foods such as confectionery – VAT. And the world is now slowly waking up to the fact that it's sugar and not fat that is implicated in obesity, heart disease, strokes, and many other things. People who still advocate a fat tax just haven't thought it through. Presumably, they don't want to tax avocados or nuts, which are both high in fat, but what happens if you sell a coated nut or preserved avocado?

Even though many people have now come to accept that sugar is bad for us, the thought still lingers in most people's minds that fat is bad also. We have not had any indication from governments or nutrition advisers that they got it wrong and that oils are not bad. Indeed we will learn later that not only is fat not bad for us but that plant and fish oils are both essential and extremely good for us.

And despite all the hype in recent decades, saturated fat isn't bad for us either and many studies over the years have shown this to be true. A recently published review summarised the results of some twenty studies that tracked over 300,000 people over 14 years, of whom some 11,000 went on to develop cardiovascular disease. They found there was no relationship whatsoever between the intake of saturated fat and the incidence of heart disease or stroke. Indeed there are several studies that now support this thesis (6,7,8,9,10).

Before we leave fats, we just need to say a few words about trans-fats, also known as hydrogenated fats. This word often crops up in the media, usually because journalists like having a poke at the food industry. The truth is that all responsible food manufacturers removed trans-fats from their products many years ago, only a short time after the realisation that these fats are not good for us. What happened was that when nutritionists proclaimed animal fats bad for us in the 70s, food manufacturers rushed to remove them from products like biscuits and cakes.

But as most housewives know, you can't successfully make a cream cake or biscuit mixes with oil, so manufacturers had to harden plant oils to make margarine and butter analogues. In doing so, about half the modified oil became trans-fat. When trans-fats in turn were declared bad, manufacturers found other ways to harden oils that did not result in high levels of trans fats, and consequently, trans fats are now old news. Just for the record, trans fats do actually occur in nature, for example, in some dairy products but generally at levels around 1 or 2% of the fat content. As often happens, I suspect that the detrimental effects of these fats have been somewhat exaggerated by parties with vested interests.

Anthropology

Anthropology is the study of man from his predecessors' time as animals.

Life has been on this earth for in excess of 3,500 million years. That is unimaginably long, so the analogy that is often used is to think of this time as one year, and on that basis, one day is equivalent to about 10 million

---

years, and so man has been on the planet for rather less than an hour. Alternatively, we can think of all that's happened in the two thousand years since Christianity began and then realise that just one million years is five hundred times that long.

Much of the chemistry involved in turning food into energy is inherited from very early times, and indeed we share a lot of it with simple bacteria living today. Until man settled down and stopped being nomadic, which coincided with the advent of farming a mere 10–12,000 years ago, he was a hunter-gatherer. So in small family groups, they hunted small animals, ate fish as they always lived by a source of freshwater, and gathered leaves and shoots that would be similar to eating salads and vegetables today.

Such a diet was rich in fibre and protein, contained roughly equal quantities of animal, plant, and fish fats, and, significantly, contained virtually no digestible carbohydrate or sugar. Significant quantities of carbohydrates only entered our ancestors' diets when man realised that he could get a lot of Calories from a small acreage of cereal and thus could stop being nomadic. So the introduction of flour and bread into our diets is a very recent phenomenon and one which 3,500 million years of biochemistry had not equipped our bodies to deal with. But the human body is very adaptable and manages to deal with carbohydrates, but it does not like them.

Worse again is sugar. Although sugar from cane arrived from the Americas in the 15th and 16th centuries, it was very expensive, and it only became available in any real quantity to the population as a whole in the last few decades of the 19th century when sugar beet was grown in Europe and sugar factories sprung up in many European countries. Significant increases in heart disease and strokes began to occur only a couple of decades after sugar became widely available.

Twenty years or so is enough for our bodies to show significant effects of a poor diet, and that was exactly what happened in the early 1900s when the incidence of heart attacks and strokes began to increase alarmingly. A few years ago, a study on teenage American army recruits found that many of them already showed evidence of significant arterial damage from poor diets, even though after their army training, they were considered fit young men (11). A handful of studies has shown that the same is true of European teenagers (12). Indeed with sophisticated methods now available, we can detect heart disease evidence in pre-school children, and there are even reports of similar problems in unborn babies because of poor eating by the mother. We need to ensure good nutrition from the very earliest years, and that is why the enormous rise in childhood obesity in recent times spells trouble for those children in later years.

More about energy for those interested.

There are four energy sources in the body.

There is a little over a heaped teaspoonful of glucose (about 9g) circulating in the 8 pints or so (4.5 litres) of blood in the adult body. This is only about 40 Calories. Glucose is the preferred energy source for the brain and red blood cells, so this level must be tightly controlled by the liver. Glucose is replenished by the food that we eat

---

or after several hours of starvation from glycogen stored in the liver. As there is only about one teaspoon of sugar in our blood, imagine how much blood sugar would rise if we eat several teaspoons worth of sugar, as in our breakfast above.

There is about one pound (half a kilogram) of glycogen in the liver and leg muscles equivalent to about 2000 Calories. Glycogen binds about twice its own weight of water, and it is therefore, only about a third as energy-dense as glucose. This glycogen is enough for about a day's energy needs if no food is eaten, and the person is mostly resting.

About 25,000 Calories of energy are stored as protein, mostly in muscle, but this is not normally used unless the person has not eaten for many days.

But in even a reasonably slim person, about 100,000 calories are stored as animal fat (about 11kg or some 16% of body weight), enough for 40–50 days of total starvation. Incidentally, if this number of Calories was stored as glycogen, which is much less Calorie dense than fat, our body weight would be about 60 kg heavier which explains why fat and not glycogen is the preferred energy source selected by evolution.

The fat is stored in specialised fat cells (adipose cells), where the fat takes up most of the cell volume. When you grill a steak or a lamb chop with a layer of fat on the outside, most of the fat melts and drips out of the cells. Left behind are the remains of the dead cells, mostly protein that, devoid of fat, becomes nice and crisp.

Finally, in this chapter, let's look at which carbohydrates raise blood sugar very rapidly and which raise it more slowly. The Glycaemic Index (GI) attempts to do this by ranking carbohydrates relative to an equal weight of glucose itself, which is given the number 100. The lower the GI of the food, the more slowly it raises blood sugar. However, the values are only approximate and depend on several factors, for example, the way foods are cooked. A boiled potato has a GI of above 90, but if you allow the potato to go cold, the GI drops to about 85. Heat it up again, and the GI drops further. Mash it with a nob of butter, and the GI drops to below 70 (the effect of butterfat).

High GI foods (70–100) include white rice, boiled and jacket potato, most commercial breakfast cereals, root vegetables such as parsnips, turnips and swede, watermelon, and most non-diet bottled fizzy drinks, sweetened fruit juices, and jams.

Moderate GI foods (50–70) include brown rice, wholemeal bread, chips, and crisps (the effect of oil), most biscuits, most confectionery bars, fruits in syrup, unsweetened fruit juices, some whole fruits including pineapple and bananas, honey, sweetcorn, and carrots.

Low GI foods (below 50) include pasta, most whole fruits (note that most fruit juices are moderate GI), and most milk and yogurt products that don't contain added sugar. Note that cheeses have no residual sugar and therefore are zero GI. So are most vegetables and salads other than those mentioned above, and meat, fish, and eggs.

What Is Natural?

A much overused word

This brings us on to what was natural for our ancestors to eat. Natural is a very over-used word these days. It is used by marketing people to elevate clearly manufactured foods to the status of foods providing great nutrition. Take "natural" apple or orange juice in a packet or bottle. Even assuming it has no added sugar, where do you find apple or orange juice in nature?

I am not being pedantic here. Even whole apples are only natural in the autumn when they ripen on the trees. You cannot naturally eat an apple in the northern hemisphere in January, February, March, April, May, June, July, August, early September or probably late November and December. Indeed, you cannot eat any fruit in temperate places other than in the autumn except by artificially "forcing" it in greenhouses or polythene tunnels or by importing it from abroad.

Nature has a very good reason for this. The purpose of fruit as far as the plant is concerned is to protect its seeds and to attract animals to eat the fruit and seeds and thus to disperse the seeds over a wide area. Therefore, over geological time, successful plants were those that kept the maximum number of animals alive during hard winters to distribute more of their seeds. So temperate plants have developed fruits that are fattening to animals because they contain large quantities of sugars. This enables the animals to put on a thick layer of fat in the autumn to help them survive a harsh winter. Fat both insulates the animal to help keep it warm and acts as an energy dense food store that can be broken down to energy and heat in the winter when food is scarce. When we well-fed humans eat fruit, we do not have periods in our life when food is scarce and our fat deposits rarely need to be called upon unless we choose to diet quite severely for a reasonably long period.

Animals and birds living in temperate places have a severe diet forced on them every winter; just look outside on a cold winter's day and you'll see trees and bushes stripped of leaves and berries and most of the insects have died leaving only their eggs or pupae to overwinter. Animals and birds really do have a severe diet forced on them every year. Robins for example typically live for about three years in the wild because many of them starve, but in captivity where they have food and warmth all year round they can live for fifteen years or longer. Even birds that choose to migrate fly thousands of miles, often without stopping and that almost totally depletes their energy stores. We humans have a very easy life these days.

Fruit juices are worse than the whole fruit, as with juice there is no flesh to contain the sugars. When we drink the juice, we are effectively drinking a solution of sugar in water. It is significant that most tropical fruits such as nuts, avocados, palms, coffee and cocoa beans are fat based and not sugar based, as animals in the tropics don't have to endure harsh winters. So in Africa, where humans evolved, there is virtually no carbohydrate for animals to eat; their diet consists almost entirely of protein, fibre and fat.

Our African ancestors would have eaten plenty of oil-based fruits. Because the tropics are warm all the time, fruit is not always very seasonal and much of it is available all year round. Even cultivated crops such as cocoa have two crops a year. So our ancestors would have had plenty of plant oils in their diet; they certainly did not eat a low-fat diet.

Of course, not all natural materials are good for us. Deadly Nightshade, yew berries and the death cap fungus (to name but a few) are extremely poisonous to humans. So natural is not necessarily good. We should not be taken in by advertisers' claims of "natural" when clearly no manufactured food can possibly be natural.

The Value of Antioxidants

Nature's damage prevention chemicals

As fruit and fruit juices contain so much sugar, why are we constantly being advised to eat plenty of fruit or to drink fruit juice? The answer is because plant material such as fruit and vegetables is very rich in antioxidants.

What are antioxidants?

Most of us know from our school science days that oxygen exists in the air around us as a molecule of two atoms of oxygen, O_2. But in the complex chemistry that goes on in our bodies, single atoms of oxygen are often produced; we could call them O_1. These free radicals, as they are known, are very unstable and very dangerous. They combine with anything they can in a tiny fraction of a second to stabilise themselves. Sometimes this is with another atom of oxygen, which forms a safe molecule of O_2.

But very often something else arrives first and this is then said to be oxidised. If this something else happens to be nucleic acid (DNA or RNA) or one of the very many other chemicals needed for cell reproduction and control, the chemical can be modified so that it no longer works

---

properly. A cell may lose the very sophisticated mechanisms that control how and when it should divide, and instead, it can begin to divide randomly and often rapidly and the familiar cancerous tumour is initiated. If our body is well supplied with antioxidants, then free radicals are much more likely to combine with the antioxidant, and cell damage is less likely to occur. Similarly, antioxidants also reduce the likelihood of arterial disease and probably many other diseases also.

There are plenty of antioxidants in low sugar-containing plant materials, such as vegetables, salads, and tropical fruits, such as nuts and seeds. Because of their high sugar content, we should consider eating temperate fruits sparingly.

Some antioxidants can occur at high levels in manufactured foods. One of the best-known antioxidants is resveratrol, which finds its way into red wine because it (unlike white wine) is fermented over grape skins where this antioxidant is concentrated. Plain (dark) chocolate contains high levels of flavonoids because cocoa beans themselves are a rich source of these antioxidants, and if you choose a chocolate (not confectionery) bar with a high cocoa solids content, the sugar levels will be low. Similarly, tomato puree and tomato sauce are rich sources of lycopene from tomatoes, and this can quite literally be a saviour to people who live on a burger diet. Vitamins A, C, and E, the so-called ACE vitamins, are also good antioxidants.

However, our bodies really do need good levels of a wide range of different antioxidants. These can only be provided by eating lots of different vegetables, salads, and fruit (this in moderation) in a wide-ranging and balanced diet. That is another reason why the sort of research described in the introduction, where single foodstuffs are promoted to be beneficial for one particular disease, is not very helpful.

So we come to the so-called five a day. But why just five? The World Health Organisation decided that 400g of vegetable material is required, divided neatly into five eighty-gram portions. And five is a number that is slightly challenging for some people but generally achievable for much of the population. Much better than the five a day mantra is to ensure that the vegetable and salad portions of your meal look just as big as the meat/fish and potato portions combined.

A mixed salad for lunch could contain lettuce (several sorts), tomato, cucumber, avocado, peppers, olives, beetroot, radishes, raw fresh peas in season, pine nuts, toasted sesame seeds, toasted pumpkin seeds, and any other salad items you can think of. Far more than five here. Stir fry for the evening meal could contain sliced carrots, broccoli, beans (several sorts), courgette, cauliflower, bean-spouts, and mange tout, to name but a few. So five a day isn't really challenging at all, which brings us to so-called "superfoods". These are foodstuffs that get a mention in the media every few months and, in the view of their exponents, work wonders. One of the latest such superfoods is turmeric that contains curcumin that appears to be quite a good anti-inflammatory. But over the last few years, we have also been told that blueberries (and other berries), chia, cranberries, edamame beans, garlic, ginger, green tea, kale, kefir, kiwifruit, mangoes, nuts, papaya, pomegranates, quinoa, shiitake mushrooms, spirulina and watermelon to name but a few are also brilliant for us.

Most of these contain weight for weight, very high levels of antioxidants, vitamins, and minerals, and can be eaten as part of a balanced diet, but not over-indulged. And the names of some of these antioxidants are bewildering; as well as those we have mentioned already, polyphenols, phytoestrogens, and chemo preventers have also been used, but the general term antioxidant covers them all.

Herbs also contain high levels of antioxidants. Rosemary will grow in any garden and is a must with lamb or new potatoes rolled in olive oil and baked in the oven. Basil will grow on any sunny windowsill if given plenty of water and can be used with almost any Italian dish. Dill will also grow on windowsills and is a must with many fish dishes. Mint and chives grow inside or out and are lovely with new potatoes. There are many others.

You might also consider choosing free-range poultry and meat from grass-fed animals because of elevated antioxidant content. It is as simple as saying that if animals get good antioxidant levels in their diet, this will be passed on to us via their meat. Several studies suggest that grass-based diets elevate precursors for Vitamin A and E and cancer-fighting antioxidants such as glutathione and superoxide dismutase. It is the antioxidant precursors of vitamin A that give corn fed poultry its yellow colour.

Cholesterol

Don't be frightened by it; it's essential for our bodies

The cell reproduction system is not the only part of our bodies that is susceptible to oxidation.

What is cholesterol?

Cholesterol is a fat that is transported around our bodies attached to proteins. The Greek word for fat is lipid, and therefore these are known as lipoproteins. There are two main types: low-density lipoprotein or LDL cholesterol is the so-called "bad" cholesterol as this moves cholesterol from the liver where it is made out to the tissues where free cholesterol can be deposited. High-density lipoprotein or HDL, the so-called "good" cholesterol, takes cholesterol from tissue back to the liver where it can be broken down.

The main concern most of us have about cholesterol is that it can block our coronary arteries. There is still much to understand about the precise mechanism of cholesterol deposition. However, in general, cholesterol seems to be deposited if the LDL-cholesterol bond is oxidised (that word again). This oxidised LDL is taken up by a type of immune system cell (macrophages) that

---

become bloated and form foam cells. Foam cells are trapped in the artery walls and contribute to the formation of plaque. Antioxidants play a vital role in preventing this oxidation. They reduce the deposition of cholesterol in the coronary arteries that take blood to the heart muscle and in the carotid arteries that take blood to the brain. Of course, it is deposits in the coronary and carotid arteries that contribute to angina, heart attacks, and strokes.

Despite its reputation as a bad guy, cholesterol is absolutely essential to our bodies.

1. It is required in cell membranes where together with unsaturated fats, it helps to keep the membrane flexible and prevents the cell from bursting. There are in excess of thirty trillion cells in our bodies, and each one has an outer membrane. There are also membranes around internal cell structures such as the nucleus and mitochondria, where energy is generated and a complex membrane skeleton in each cell, which gives the cell its shape and ensures each substance goes to the right place in the cell. So membranes are vitally important in the body, and cholesterol (and unsaturated fats) are vital components of them.

2. Cholesterol is an essential component of bile, which is secreted into the small intestine and helps us digest fats. Without bile, fats cannot be made water-soluble and absorbed into the body.

3. Cholesterol is an essential component of the myelin sheaths of nerves, and without cholesterol, our nerves may simply not work properly.

4. But perhaps most importantly, cholesterol is an essential starting point in the synthesis of the five major classes of steroid hormones. You will probably have heard of many of these: progestogens (such as progesterone), glucocorticoids (such as cortisol), mineralocorticoids (that assist kidney function), androgens (such as testosterone), and oestrogens (that participate in the ovarian cycle). Our bodies convert sterols such as cholesterol into sterones such as proge*sterone* and testo*sterone*. Without cholesterol, these sex hormones could not be synthesized, none of us would be here, and indeed, the animal kingdom could not have advanced as it has done.

So far from being bad for us, cholesterol is absolutely essential. Adults need about 1.5–2.0 grams of cholesterol (about a third of a teaspoon) per day for these functions, about half of which is provided by a normal omnivorous diet (vegetarians and particularly vegans obviously ingest significantly less).

A common misunderstanding is that we can reduce cholesterol levels in our blood by reducing our dietary cholesterol. Unfortunately, many food companies promote their products as low cholesterol in an attempt to deceive us into thinking they will lower our cholesterol. They will not. Our bodies can make cholesterol in the liver, and our bodies can break down cholesterol so that if we eat less cholesterol, the body just makes more. Biochemists have known this for decades, but advice just hasn't caught up. As recently as a few years ago, do you remember being told that we mustn't eat more than three eggs a week as they contain lots of cholesterol? And perhaps you've noticed that this very bad advice has just disappeared. We have had no apology for having been steered away from eggs, which are one of the best and cheapest sources of protein generally available to all of us.

I first became interested in nutrition some 35 years ago when I went for a cholesterol test. The result was high. I was given the usual diet sheet, which advised cutting out all the culprits normally blamed, such as red meat, dairy products, eggs, and general fat. I followed this regime slavishly for three months and went for a repeat test in the total belief that my blood cholesterol would have fallen considerably. It hadn't budged. It was exactly the same as it had been three months earlier. When I mentioned this to the nurse who took the blood, she just shrugged. When I mentioned this to a number of friends, many had had similar experiences and, indeed, I have met very many people today and over the intervening years who have had similar experiences. It seemed that there was something wrong with the "science".

The truth is that it seems extremely difficult to reduce cholesterol with diet alone. One of the few ways of doing so is to consume cholesterol analogues in the form of plant sterols and stanols that fool the body into thinking that it has more cholesterol than it actually has. Plant stanols are now added to some dairy products such as spreads and yogurts.

Much has also been written about statins as a means of reducing cholesterol. Most of the research into statins and cholesterol has been done either directly by pharmaceutical companies or has been sponsored by them. What is correct is basic science.

Cholesterol science simplified

Our coronary arteries that feed the heart muscle with blood are quite small; they have an internal diameter little bigger than a pencil lead. During our lives, these vessels can become coated internally with plaque that does indeed contain cholesterol amongst many other components.

These deposits have the dual effect of narrowing the arteries and making the arterial walls less flexible so that they are less able to widen and contract again with each pulse of blood. Narrowing of these coronary arteries reduces blood flow to the heart, and during periods of exercise may result in the familiar chest pain called angina.

However, what is worse is that if even a small blood clot arrives at a point where the artery is narrowed, the clot may become lodged by the plaque and may immediately shut off the supply of blood to the heart along that artery, and the heart may stop; a heart attack.

As explained above, high levels of antioxidants reduce the likelihood that LDL cholesterol will be oxidised and significantly reduce deposition, narrowing, and a consequent arterial blockage.

Hardening of arteries may also occur. Blood flow through the arteries is not constant, as is the flow of water through a hosepipe. It pulses with each beat of the heart. Cholesterol deposits can reduce the artery wall's ability to expand and contract with each pulse of blood. If this happens in the aorta, the main artery taking blood from the heart, it may burst with a strong pulse of blood, and an aneurysm occurs, a major bleed into the chest or abdominal cavity that may well be fatal. An aneurysm can also occur in the brain and is another cause of strokes.

Smaller arteries and veins can also get blocked or burst, but the effect is often less dramatic and may not even be noticed as the body often finds alternative routes to get blood to body extremities.

Remember also the benefits of exercise. We should aim to do some form of brisk exercise for half an hour or so, at least every other day. Examples of such exercise include a brisk walk or gentle run, swimming, playing a sport such as football or tennis or going to the gym.

But just like eating, exercise should be fun, otherwise we will soon stop doing it. There is no need to do strenuous heavy exercises such as running marathons or weight lifting. Such exercise may put undue stress on the body, particularly if we're not used to it. Remember anthropology: we wandered around all day scavenging for food and heavy exercise was confined to short bursts of sprinting to catch animal food or to escape predators.

Although regular exercise does not significantly change the total cholesterol level in our bodies, it does raise the proportion of HDL, the "good" cholesterol. In top athletes, the proportion of HDL can approach 50% of the total blood cholesterol, whereas in couch potatoes, it may be below 10% of the total. Smoking tobacco is also known to reduce the proportion of HDL cholesterol and increase LDL oxidation leading to cholesterol deposits.

I believe that provided we have high antioxidant levels in our bodies, the detrimental effects of elevated blood cholesterol have been overstated. Taking myself as an example, the only time I have used the Health Service (other than for my annual routine check-up) was when I deliberately went for a few heart checks a few years ago. I didn't have a problem; I just wanted to see whether my continued high blood cholesterol levels were having any ill effects. They could find no evidence of any build-up in my coronary or carotid arteries, nor in my aorta. Yet I have had elevated blood cholesterol now for at least the last thirty-five years and I have not taken statins. I would rather have natural cholesterol in my body than an artificial chemical. I take the view that if the healthy body has that level of cholesterol, it is because it needs it. In my case, because I eat more fat than most people, I need more bile to help break it down. That means more cholesterol than most people and thus my own cholesterol levels are relatively high (15).

A much better marker for coronary heart disease in my view is triglyceride (TG), which is a fat that circulates in the blood. Remember that blood fats are made from sugar and that diets high in sugar often result in high blood triglyceride levels. Doctors normally measure this at the same time as a cholesterol test is done, but the results are sometimes overlooked. Blood triglyceride should be low, and unlike cholesterol, it is easy to control it both by lowering dietary sugar and in another way that I will explain later in the chapter on fats.

Milk and Dairy Products

Can nature's full-fat milk really be bad for us?

As well as eggs, we have been told repeatedly that full-fat milk and full fat dairy products are bad for us. We are urged to use watery, low-fat options.

Yet how can this be? After all, milk is produced by mothers to feed and nourish their offspring, and nature surely does not gratuitously harm its young. Yes, cow's milk is a little different in composition and richer than human milk, but it's not that different. Human milk is generally a little lower in protein than cows' milk but is higher in lactose.

Milk is the perfect, virtually complete food. It has almost equal quantities of protein, only slowly fermentable carbohydrate and fat, and is rich in minerals and vitamins. It lacks iron because the mother has used substantial amounts of iron in growing the baby, and vitamin C, because vitamin C is acidic (ascorbic acid) and it could curdle the milk. Yet again, it seems that the only reason we're told to reduce our intake of dairy products is because they contain cholesterol. Yet we have already seen that cholesterol is required for healthy tissue and is only dangerous if we don't get plenty of antioxidant through eating a diet rich in vegetables and salads.

Surely if our mother's milk feeds us cholesterol, it can hardly be harmful to us. Mothers don't harm their offspring. The use of skimmed and semi-skimmed milk rather than whole milk has two disadvantages. Firstly, it is known that sugars are absorbed much more quickly in the absence of fat. Foods that contain mixtures of fats and sugars such as whole milk, flour confectionery, chocolate, and ice-cream result in blood sugar rising more slowly than an equivalent amount of sugar on its own, for example, in a fizzy drink. Secondly, there is virtually no fat in skimmed milk to coat the intestinal wall, and thus, more calories and more sugar are absorbed and absorbed more quickly than with whole milk.

Because milk is the most natural and complete food there is, we can base our diet in later life on its components. We should consider eating roughly equal quantities of fat, protein, and slowly fermentable carbohydrate as in whole milk. Much of the carbohydrate can be replaced after infancy with fibre, which newly born intestines would be unable to digest. The sugar in milk is lactose that the infant body breaks down slowly to a mixture of glucose and another sugar called galactose, which is not fermented and therefore does not raise blood sugar. Glucose is released only at about the rate that the baby's body needs it for energy.

The fat content of milk is also interesting. It is almost two-thirds saturated fat, about one-quarter monounsaturated fat, and less than 5% polyunsaturated fat (the significance of this will be seen over the next two chapters). If these were not ideal ratios for our bodies, nature would have developed milk differently over the millions of years that mammals have been on earth. The saturated fat in milk is soft (as in butter) so that it's easier for infants to digest than harder forms of saturated fat found in meat. It is also interesting that milk contains an unusual fat called CLA (conjugated linoleic acid) that is thought to be beneficial to the heart and blood (13,14).

Also, in the fat layer are emulsifiers such as lecithin that retard the separation of the fat from the water. Emulsifiers are good for our bodies as they perform exactly the same function there, helping fats to mix with water in blood, for example. If you drink only skimmed milk, you are missing out on these components.

The solids content of milk is about 12%, so some 88% of it is water. This is close to the ideal ratio for the adult body also. Most of us not on a diet eat between 1350 and 1800g (3–4 lbs) of food during a typical day. A proportion of this will be water, typically 50–60% in raw meat and fish, 70–80% in fruit and vegetables but rather less after cooking, and considerably less in processed and baked goods. In order to increase our total water intake to close that in milk, we need to drink some two to three litres (four to five pints) of liquid, and more if it's a hot day. I suspect that most of us don't come close to that figure and are therefore in danger of dehydration. Early in the morning is a critical time as we lose quite a lot of liquid overnight.

And, of course, if you eat more, you will also need to drink more.

Fantastic Fats

It's the sugar that's the problem, not fats

What causes blood to form dangerous clots that can block narrowed arteries? This is not the same mechanism that causes blood to form a scab if the skin is cut or grazed. Arterial blood clots occur when the smallest of the blood corpuscles called platelets aggregate together. Platelet agglomeration is more likely to occur when platelets become "sticky," and this, in turn, is controlled by lovely chemicals with very long and difficult names, so we'll simply call them signalling chemicals. The chemistry of these (which just for biochemists are the eicosanoids that include prostaglandins, prostacyclins, thromboxanes, and leucotrines) and their mechanism of control is extremely complex and not entirely understood, but I will try to simplify everything, although I am sure researchers in this area may take issue with some of the over-simplification.

In essence, there are two main series of these signalling chemicals.

Series 2 is derived from certain types of plant oils, the polyunsaturated oils, sometimes called omega-6 oils.

Series 3 is derived from fish oils or so-called omega-3 oils.

These two series of signalling chemicals work together synergistically and also against one another antagonistically. So, for example, Series 2 increases platelet aggregation. In contrast, Series 3 reduces "stickiness." The amount of "stickiness" will largely depend on the relative amounts of the relevant Series 2 and Series 3 signalling chemicals in our bodies. If our bodies contain a lot of polyunsaturated plant oil, our blood will be more "sticky" than if we have recently consumed fish.

But these signalling chemicals also control lots of other things. For example, blood pressure is increased by high levels of Series 2 but decreased by high levels of Series 3. And inflammation, particularly ongoing chronic inflammation, can be promoted by high levels of polyunsaturates. To help understand, let's tabulate this.

	Series 2 Plant oil (polyunsaturated)	Series 3 Fish oil
Platelet clotting	Increases	Reduces
Blood pressure	Increases	Reduces
Inflammation	Increases	Reduces

This helps to explain why heart disease, strokes, and high blood pressure were almost unknown in traditional fish-eating communities such as Japan and Greenland. Fish oils (so-called omega-3 oils) are also good for the eyes (including the prevention of cataracts, glaucoma, and ocular hypertension), the brain (they may benefit several psychiatric disorders including depression), rhinitis and the reduction of mucus production, the immune system, and they also lower blood triglyceride (in conjunction with a low sugar diet). Their value can hardly be over-emphasised. Unfortunately, these signalling chemicals are very short-lived in the body (typically seconds) and so we must ensure the correct ratios of fats in the body at all times.

However, we must bear in mind that fish don't make fish oil. Like us, fish are animals and would make animal fat except that there is virtually no carbohydrate in the sea from which to make it. Fatty fish such as salmon, trout, and mackerel accumulate the oil in their tissues from a lifetime of feeding on plankton, krill, and in particular on blue-green algae in cold oceanic waters. If you eat farmed fish, the fish will contain oils from what the fish-farmer feeds them. In the early days of fish farming, food such as millet was used that contains almost exclusively plant omega-6 oils. These days many fish-farmers are aware of this and make an attempt to use omega-3 oils, although in many cases, this is omega-3 oil derived from certain plants such as linseed and flax. Although omega-3, these vegetable oils are fundamentally different from fish oil and not as good for us. Plant omega-3 is only about 5% as effective as fish omega-3 in the human body, so we need twenty times as much plant omega-3 oil to have the same effect. This is a concern for vegetarians and vegans, but the rest of us should eat wild fish wherever possible.

This is also an issue for conservation as wild fish stocks are at low levels almost worldwide. Whitefish also consume large quantities of oil from plankton, but they store this oil in the liver. So their flesh is relatively low in fish oil. Livers from white fish such as cod are used to make bottled oil and oil in capsules, but the whole livers are extremely high in vitamin A which is toxic in high concentration, so don't be tempted to eat fish liver. However, fish livers are a possible solution to the problem of where to get good quality omega-3 oils without over-fishing.

Krill is a tiny marine shrimp that feeds on blue-green algae, and some people state that krill oil is better for us than fish oil. This is partly because it is very rich in an antioxidant called astaxanthin. As we can get antioxidants from many plant sources, it is probably better to preserve krill stocks and not to upset the delicate marine ecosystem.

Remember that if you take fish oil or cod liver oil or similar, you should keep it in the fridge and away from light. Freshly caught fish is not fishy, but immediately it is landed, the oil begins to oxidise (that word again), and chemicals called cyclic peroxides are formed. Not only do these taste fishy (as fish several days' old does) but they are not good for us. And unfortunately, the oil in fish oil capsules also oxidises over time as the gelatine capsule is not an oxygen barrier, so keep capsules in the fridge also. Oxidation is over ten times slower at refrigeration temperatures than it is at room temperature.

However, let's not forget plant oils. We saw above that polyunsaturated oils can increase inflammation. Monounsaturated oils do not. We will examine these further in the next chapter. But for now, let's remember what we learnt about membranes in the chapter on cholesterol. Membranes surround every cell in our body and protect and enclose many of the cell's internal structures. As well as cholesterol, membranes are rich in unsaturated fats. And although, as we know, the body can make cholesterol, it cannot make unsaturated oils. It is vital that we get plenty of unsaturated plant oils in our diet to keep the cell membrane flexible, prevent it from breaking and causing the cell to die, and allow the membrane to function correctly. Membranes allow things that the cell needs to enter but keeps out things that it doesn't want. And many cells have short life spans, so to make new membranes, the body needs a constant supply of good quality plant oils.

Plant oils also oxidise, although much more slowly than fish oils. Hydroperoxides are formed that change into aldehydes that give oils the familiar rancid taste. This is not a problem when the bottle is full as there is very little headspace and thus not much oxygen but if you use the oil only slowly, consider keeping that in the fridge.

Inflammation

Chronic inflammation is a sign that things aren't right

In the previous chapter, we learned that inflammation was controlled, at least in part, by signalling chemicals and that polyunsaturated plant oils increase chronic inflammation, whereas fish oil reduces it.

Inflammation manifests itself in many ways. Skin rashes, skin irritability and eczema, hay fever and pollen allergies, asthma, arthritis, and hypersensitivity to a wide range of foodstuffs are all manifestations of inflammation. More recently, many other diseases are claimed to have an inflammation element, for example, heart disease, cancer, and Alzheimer's disease.

We often ask why so many more people seem to have allergies today compared with a few decades ago, and this is often dismissed with the glib answer that people back then weren't as aware of these ailments as they are today. I doubt that is true; people would have been equally concerned about these effects on their bodies as we are today. One of the main reasons why inflammation is so prevalent today is the huge growth in our intake of polyunsaturated plant oils over the last four or five decades.

Remember that anthropology tells us that the ratio of animal to plant to fish oils in diets has traditionally been about the same (1:1:1), whereas over the last 40–50 years the level of plant oil consumption has increased to ten or even twenty times that of animal and fish oils (17). Therefore, it follows that we should be able to reverse allergies by reducing our intake of polyunsaturated oils substantially from plants and increasing the level of fish oil in our diet. However, this is not a quick fix. Suppose we weigh 75kg and our body fat content is 20%. This means that we have 15kg or 15,000g of fat in our bodies. Even if we take 5g of cod liver oil per day, it will take a long time to flush out all of the excess plant oil that we have consumed during our lives.

More about fats for those interested

Fats (fatty acids) comprise a chain of carbon atoms. The chains can be short (4–8) as in milk, as these fats, being slightly soluble in water, are easily digested by infants. Medium length chains (12–18) are the most common in plants and animals. Long chains (20–22) are found in fish, and their food sources blue-green algae, plankton, and krill.

Attached to each carbon is hydrogen, and when each carbon has as much hydrogen as it can take, the fat is said to be **saturated** with hydrogen. These, of course, are the principal components of animal fat.

If one or more carbons loses some of its hydrogens, the fat becomes **unsaturated** with hydrogen or dehydrogenated. Just doing this turns a solid fat into oil. In nature, this process begins at carbon number 9, and if this is the only carbon that loses its hydrogen, the oil is said to be **monounsaturated or omega-9.** These are the principal components of monounsaturated oils such as olive oil and rapeseed oil.

If two or more carbons lose some of their hydrogens, the oil is said to be **polyunsaturated.** As well as carbon number 9, carbon number 6 is the next to become unsaturated, and therefore these oils are known as **omega-6.** These are the principal components of polyunsaturated plant oils such as sunflower, corn, and safflower oils.

The third carbon to become unsaturated in nature (in addition to 9 and 6) is number 3, and these oils are known as **omega-3.** Two omega-3 oils occur in some plants, and these are known as ALA and GLA. ALA (alpha-linolenic acid) occurs in high levels in linseed and carmelina oils and in lower quantities in, amongst others, rapeseed, soybean, and wheat germ oils, blackcurrant seeds, and walnuts. GLA (gamma-linolenic acid) is the active ingredient in evening primrose and borage oils said to help with ladies' ailments.

The long-chained omega-3 oils occur only in marine food sources. These are far superior for our bodies than the plant omega-3 oils and are used to make Series 3 controllers as described in the last chapter.

Trans fats are those where the hydrogen is lost from the opposite sides of adjacent carbons, whereas in cis fats, hydrogen is lost from the same side. Cis are the unsaturated fats that predominate in nature, although there are small quantities of naturally occurring trans fats, for example, in milk.

Finally, these fatty acids are not normally transported and stored in this form. Fats are insoluble in water, and since the body is an aqueous medium, fats have to be converted into a soluble form. This is done in the body by attaching the fatty acids to glycerine (glycerol), which is a sweet, colourless, and moderately thick liquid that you can buy from pharmacies. The glycerine molecule is shaped like the letter E, and a fatty acid attaches itself to each of the three bars of the E to form a triglyceride. Remember that triglycerides are formed in the blood from excess sugar and are often measured by doctors at the same time as cholesterol.

And just for the record, cholesterol itself has a very different, complicated ring structure containing 27 carbon atoms.

Inflammation and the common cold

Nutrition can affect the aetiology of the common cold and quite possibly other viral diseases such as influenza. When you have a cold, many people take preparations containing aspirin or paracetamol. These work by reducing inflammation, which they do by manipulating our signalling chemicals as described earlier. So reduced inflammation in our brain reduces headaches, reduced inflammation in our throats and lungs lessens sore throats and coughing, and reduced inflammation in our sinuses reduces blocked and runny noses.

But if we eat toast for breakfast smothered with a polyunsaturated spread or indeed other polyunsaturated containing foods, we are increasing the very signalling chemicals that increase inflammation. These fight against aspirin or paracetamol and consequently, these preparations are not as effective as they would have been had we not eaten these polyunsaturates.

The signalling chemicals made from plant and fish oils exert important control on the immune system. With nearly perfect balance, I have found it possible to avoid colds and flu. I have not had flu for over thirty years, even though my lifestyle means I'm often exposed to it.

So what are the best fats and oils to eat and the worst? The following table shows approximate levels of monounsaturates, polyunsaturates and saturates in a number of common oils and fats. There can be quite a lot of variation in these natural materials so these are typical values. Those oils at the top of the table have the lowest polyunsaturate content.

It is interesting that butter and indeed human milk contain very low levels of polyunsaturated fat.

	Monounsaturate	Polyunsaturates	Saturates
Macadamia Nut	82	2	14
Butter	22	3	52
Olive	65	12	17
Lard	45	11	43
Hazelnut	77	12	9
Avocado	71	15	14
Linseed*	20	15	4
Rapeseed**	70	18	5
Almond	70	21	8
Peanut	46	32	17

Brazil Nut	40	35	25
Soybean	28	50	14
Corn Oil	28	55	13
Wheat Germ	28	54	15
Walnut	30	58	10
Grapeseed	24	65	10
Sunflower	16	72	11
Safflower	7	76	17

*Note that linseed oil contains a substantial quantity (about 55%) of ALA (alpha-linolenic acid), which is the most common plant omega-3 oil. **Rapeseed and soybean oils contain about 8% and wheat germ oil, about 3%. Values may not always add to 100% because there are other components also, including up to 1% water. Butter contains around 20% water.

From soybean and below, the amount of polyunsaturates exceeds the amount of monounsaturates, and we should consider not using too much of these oils. Also, we should not use these oils for frying as polyunsaturates are not as stable to heat as monounsaturates and particularly saturates are, and chemical changes occur with heat that can produce chemicals (aldehydes) that have been linked to cancer. Therefore, don't use these oils in deep-fat frying where the oil is often used repeatedly and only topped up with fresh oil as necessary. Unfortunately, this is often the case in many fast-food outlets and restaurants where chips are served. Chefs like polyunsaturated oils like sunflower oil as they are lighter and cheaper than monounsaturates or butter, but we should always use butter, lard, olive or rapeseed for health reasons for frying and keep cooking temperatures as low as possible and certainly not allow the fat to smoke.

It is also good to choose cold-pressed oils over cheaper brands that are usually extracted by heat. For example, olives are rich in tocopherols related to vitamin E and toco-trienols, both of which are excellent antioxidants. Cold-pressed olive oil, particularly extra virgin, is rich in these components, whereas the high temperatures used in heat extracted oils destroy most of these valuable antioxidants. The better oils are sold in dark glass bottles as all oils are affected by light to some extent and, over time, begin to turn rancid, particularly as the oil is used and air introduced into the bottle. These days many supermarkets sell avocado oil, hazelnut oil, or other nut oils, so try cooking with some of these or using them in dressings to vary the flavour.

Brilliant Bacteria

Only a few are bad; many are essential

Some scientists think that many of the allergies we have today may be because bacteria are not frequently challenging our immune system. Our lives today are simply too clean. We see advertising for cleaning and sterilising agents that depict bacteria as nasty looking creepy crawlies that only their product will destroy. Consequently, we clean all surfaces and utensils in our kitchens and our toilets and bathrooms to within an inch of their lives. This can be with products that claim to kill 99.9% of household germs. But consider that on many surfaces, a million bacteria may not be uncommon so even after 99.9% are killed, 1000 still remain!

Our immune systems need to be challenged with bacteria to keep them in good shape. Some of us will have taken holidays in south-east Asian countries, and many of us will probably have suffered from food poisoning whilst we were there. Yet the locals who are exposed to these bacteria all the time don't have problems.

What are bacteria?

Bacteria are small creatures with just one cell. If you magnify a bacterium a thousand times, it would be about the size of a full stop on this page. If you magnified a person a thousand times, he or she would be about six times the height of the Eiffel Tower. Imagine a massive structure going six thousand feet – over a mile – into the air and imagine how many full stops you could get on or in that structure.

As bacteria are so small, they occur in huge mind-boggling numbers. As I haven't cleaned my teeth for a few hours, there could well be more bacteria in my mouth than there are people in the world. And quite possibly a million times that number (several trillion) in my intestines – about four pounds or two kilograms by weight.

Because they are so small, they can multiply extremely quickly. Where there is plenty of food, water, and warmth, as in our bodies, a bacterium can divide into two about every fifteen minutes. So in an hour, one bacterium can give rise to sixteen, and if you do the arithmetic, one bacterium becomes a million in just five hours.

On the other hand, if there is no water or food, as on a dry, clean kitchen worktop, the bacterium cannot grow at all, although that doesn't necessarily mean that it will die either. And their growth is slowed considerably under refrigeration conditions and stopped entirely in a deep freeze.

Most bacteria are perfectly harmless, and for all sorts of reasons we couldn't exist without them. For example, in ruminants such as cows and rabbits, bacteria digest most of the grass and vegetation that they eat. In our intestines, bacteria also help us to digest our food and may assist in breaking down sugars quickly, which they use themselves as food and so slow our blood glucose from rising as quickly as it might have done if they weren't there. Mice can be grown aseptically, that is, without any bacteria in or on their bodies. Such mice are always weak individuals, smaller than their normally developed siblings but also seem to suffer from depression and anxiety. It seems that bacteria can synthesise many of the neurotransmitters (chemicals such as serotonin) found in our brains, which might mean that we need to look no further than optimising our gut bacteria to treat a range of mental health issues (16).

Many of the mental health and anxiety issues that have come to the fore in recent years could probably have been avoided if people had done some exercise in the fresh air every day and looked after their gut bacteria by eating fresh salads and vegetables. It is never too late to start. It is much better to try that than to run to the doctor for pills that you may end up having to take for the rest of your life.

So we need to look after our gut bacteria. The way to do this is not to waste money on expensive products claiming to contain good bacteria (many of which will be destroyed by our stomach acid on the way down). Such products usually contain only one or at most a few sorts of bacteria. A healthy gut contains perhaps a hundred different species with five to ten predominating, and by eating plenty of fresh uncooked food such as salads, nuts, or fruit, we are encouraging the whole spectrum of bacteria. If we eat only prepared ready meals, baked products, and the like that are cooked to destroy nearly all bacteria, then our intestinal flora will suffer.

Healthy individuals need only wash soiled kitchen worktops with a damp cloth and then dry them and not waste money on expensive disinfectants and sterilisers. Bacteria cannot grow without water. However, high-risk individuals whose immune systems may be compromised should, of course, take every precaution to avoid infection. In this regard, toilet lids should always be closed before flushing as this creates aerosols so that faecal bacteria can find their way onto bathroom items such as toothbrushes.

Whilst on the subject of microorganisms, let's take a quick look at viruses, moulds, and yeasts.

What are viruses?

Viruses are not generally considered living creatures. Outside their host they are completely inert. They consist only of a piece of nucleic acid (DNA or RNA) surrounded by a protein coat, the capsid. The capsid serves both to protect the DNA or RNA inside and importantly to attach the virus particle to the host cell and assist the entry of the DNA or RNA into the host. Once inside, this nucleic acid can switch off the normal functioning of the cell and cause the cell chemistry to make many copies of the virus DNA or RNA and many copies of the protein coat. The two are assembled, the cell dies and bursts open, releasing many, often hundreds of virus particles. As many cells are infected, several thousand virus particles are coughed or sneezed out of the body to affect other individuals.

> Because viruses are not free-living, they are completely unaffected by antibiotics, so there is absolutely no point in taking antibiotics for colds, flu, and childhood viral diseases such as chickenpox and measles unless the weakened body immune system allows secondary bacterial infections such as bronchitis to occur.

Viruses are not generally a problem in foodstuffs, although they can cause food poisoning if seafood such as oysters and other shellfish carrying certain viruses are consumed uncooked.

What are moulds?

Moulds are fungi that grow as filaments; hence they often look like cotton wool. They grow under dry conditions, so are often found on bread, jam, and cheese that are too dry to support bacterial growth. Moulds easily and quickly form spores that are released into the air.

Many moulds are completely harmless. White filamentous moulds (such as Mucor) can simply be cut off bread or removed from the jam and the remaining contents eaten.

However, moulds that are deeply coloured blue, black or dark grey (such as some *Penicillium* and *Aspergillus* species) can produce mycotoxins. Mycotoxins were originally identified when cattle died from ergotism after eating mouldy hay and have subsequently been shown to be carcinogenic. It is known that mycotoxins are not produced under acid conditions, such as in jams and cheese, so blue cheeses are perfectly safe. However, in non-acid foods such as bread, mycotoxins can diffuse quite some way into mouldy foodstuffs, so the safest thing is not to consume such foods at all but to dispose of them without breathing any of the spores that may be released.

Yeasts are very similar to some moulds, and indeed some moulds can grow as yeasts under certain conditions. Yeasts have, of course, been used for thousands of years to produce bread, beer, and wines, and in certain parts of the world, such as eastern Europe, fermented milk foods such as yoghurts.

Finally, in this chapter, let's just look at a few things we can do to help prevent food poisoning.

The flesh of meat or fish is sterile except on cut surfaces, which could have been contaminated by knives, hands, or similar. So provided the entire exposed surface is heated by the grill or pan, you will not get food poisoning from meat that is cooked only rare. However, this does not apply to items such as burgers and sausages made from minced or comminuted meats where all the internal surfaces may have been contaminated. These should always be cooked right through.

However, be very careful with poultry, where the central cavity will have been contaminated with bacteria from the animal's intestines when it was gutted. This cavity takes a long time to get hot, so do make sure that the juices always run clear before eating. The same applies to fish flesh adjacent to the gutted area.

And of course, avoid undercooked shellfish, eggs, and unpasteurised milk and cheeses. Make sure also that you don't transfer bacteria from dirty utensils and uncooked meat to clean utensils and food that won't be cooked.

Before we finish with bacteria, we need to mention a particularly nasty one that has the equally nasty name of *Pyphoromonas gingivalis.* This lives in the mouth, but with poor oral hygiene, it can enter the body via the gap between the teeth and the gums. It can evade the normal body defences and travel around the body in the blood. It has been associated with pericarditis (inflammation of the membrane around the heart), with some forms of dementia and with rheumatoid arthritis. That is not to say that it causes these diseases; proving cause and effect is notoriously difficult, but it may do, or it may alter the progress of these diseases. Maintaining good oral hygiene at all times and in particular, avoiding gum disease and gingivitis is very important.

Not So Brilliant Chemicals

Keep a wary eye out

Many chemicals find their way into our foods. Some are traditional and have been used for centuries. Wood smoke used to smoke salmon, trout and ham contain various chemicals that vary somewhat depending on the wood used. Hams contain salt, nitrates, and nitrites for preservation, which have been linked to cancer and other diseases in recent years. Chemical fertilisers are often added to the soil in which vegetables and salads are grown. Chemical sprays can be used to control insect pests and other diseases in the plant material we eat.

Although thorough tests are carried out on these fertilisers and insecticides to show that they are safe when used as directed, we are at the farmer's mercy to ensure that they are used at the correct concentration. At the very least, we must soak and wash all fruit, vegetables, and salads in plenty of water before cooking or eating. Organic produce avoids these problems, but organics' quality is sometimes not as good and the price may put off many people.

Many foods quite naturally contain small quantities of chemicals that could be extremely dangerous to our bodies if we ate large amounts of them. For example, almonds naturally contain tiny amounts of cyanide (almonds are of course quite safe to eat). Many vegetables and salads contain small amounts of chemicals known generically as alkaloids. Such chemicals are not dangerous in small amounts as our bodies are able to break these down in the liver. However, where these alkaloids occur naturally in larger amounts in plant materials that are not part of traditional foods, as in deadly nightshade, for example, the amounts consumed may overpower the liver's ability to deal with them.

Common salt is a chemical (sodium chloride) and has had a bad press because it is said to raise blood pressure. We have already seen that blood pressure is largely controlled by signalling chemicals made from fats and that with adequate levels of fish oil, blood pressure should not be a problem. In the body, sodium works in conjunction with potassium across membranes, and blood pressure is raised as much by low dietary potassium as by high sodium. All gardeners know that if you want to have high yields and good quality vegetables and salads, potash (potassium sulphate) must be used to fertilise the soil. Thus, vegetables and salads contain good levels of potassium. Again, salt is only likely to be a significant issue for those with poor diets.

The calls for a sugar tax will undoubtedly result in increased use of artificial sweeteners, particularly in fizzy drinks. Whilst permitted sweeteners have gone through all the EU, American, and other safety protocols, the concern does persist in some quarters about the extensive use of these sweeteners over a lifetime that is clearly beyond the ability of testing protocols to predict.

So perhaps we should return to good old-fashioned tea and coffee without sugar, and let's not forget that these both contain useful levels of antioxidants. So indeed do a large number of fruit infusions now available. Whilst some people may persist in the view that caffeine is a stimulant, it is a very mild one, and we have been consuming tea and coffee for centuries without ill-effects. And, of course, there's also good old water.

This brings us to that other chemical, alcohol. I'm sure most of us are tired of turning on the radio or television to learn that the safe limits for alcohol consumption have been lowered yet again. Such low levels are unrealistic, as people just won't keep to them. Some pundits even recommend becoming teetotal, which is even more unrealistic for most people.

We all know that if we drink on an empty stomach, we feel tipsy more quickly than if we drink with food. Drinking wine (or other alcohol such as beer or cider) with food is the best way to drink alcohol. As with sugar, absorption is much slower, and the detrimental effects less severe.

It is probably best to avoid neat high proof spirits such as shots altogether as these have been linked to oral and throat cancers. Always drink spirits such as gin or whisky with mixers or water to dilute the spirit.

Acrylamides, which have also been linked to cancer, can form during high-temperature cooking from a reaction between protein and sugars, so don't overcook foods or eat food that has been burnt during frying or grilling.

And much has also been written about plasticisers that are used to soften plastic bottles. They have been linked, amongst other things to premature balding. To be on the safe side consume drinks and milk only from glass bottles.

E numbers have received a very bad press over several decades, even though they are only given to additives that have passed EU testing regimes. Despite that, there seems little doubt that some colours such as tartrazine and sunset yellow made from coal tar (both legal in the US also) cause hyperactivity, particularly in children. Clearly, the testing regimes don't cover everything, partly because there is not always a clear understanding of how such chemicals are metabolised in the body over the period of a lifetime. Back to biochemistry again! I am not saying that all E numbers are bad for us. Some such as lecithin E322 are simply extracts of naturally occurring soya beans. But suppose you're not happy eating so many of these E numbers. In that case, the simple way to avoid them is to eat fewer ready meals and manufactured products and keep to using only the very best raw ingredients you can find cooked in simple and traditional ways. After all, the best restaurants strive to do that and done at home, it is often cheaper than buying ready meals.

Finally, the natural browning of fruit after a few days is perfectly safe. It is simply the oxidation of polyphenols in the fruit to polyquinones, so whilst unsightly it will not harm you.

Food for Our Skin

We don't only eat through our mouths

We often forget that our skin is the largest organ in the body. It covers about twenty square feet and can account for more than 20% of body weight. But it also absorbs up to 60% of the lotions and potions that we rub on to it. This is a potential issue with both men's and ladies' cosmetics.

Many of us tend to splash out on expensive perfumes, eau de toilettes, and aftershaves bought from airport duty-free shops, spending £50 or €100 on contents that often cost no more than a few pence and expensive packaging that costs a pound or three. The rest goes to the manufacturer, wholesaler, retailer, and the airport authority.

There is almost always no ingredient list, but if there were, we would shudder at the nasty chemicals we are putting on our skin. In light of this, it seems strange that, on the one hand, there is rightly substantial legislation to control the contents and manufacture of pharmaceuticals and foods, whilst on the other hand, there is relatively little legislation for cosmetics. For example, microbeads that get washed down the drains and ultimately back to rivers, seas and oceans can get eaten by fish and thus find their way back into the food chain. Most of the chemicals permitted in cosmetics are not part of the natural food chain.

Many eaux-de-Cologne, perfumes and aftershaves contain alcohols that are quite astringent and other chemicals that can cause allergic skin reactions. It's much nicer to use a soothing oil-based preparation. After all, many cosmetic creams are based on fats (the cosmetic industry likes to call them butters) and oils, but it's much nicer and considerably cheaper to blend them to your own liking. Remember also that most oils have an element of sun protection factor in them, usually around 15–20.

This is not a book about cosmetics, but here are a few thoughts.

How to make cosmetic oils

Firstly, you need a carrier oil into which you can add small quantities of aromatherapy oils.

Perhaps the most commonly used carrier oil is grapeseed oil, but this contains about 10% saturates and is, therefore, not as thin and quickly absorbed as macadamia oil. The latter is also very low in polyunsaturates, and so is not at all inflammatory. Apricot kernel, almond, and jojoba are also good carrier oils, being low in both saturate and polyunsaturates.

You can add a few drops of an aromatherapy oil of your choice.

Ladies can use combinations of Rose Otto (which is better than Rose Absolute that is solvent extracted), Ylang-Ylang, Jasmine and any of the citrus oils such as orange and lemon lime, mandarin or grapefruit.

Men might like Sandlewood or Cedarwood (both have that familiar woody aroma). Patchouli, which has a particularly pleasant heady spice aroma, is reputedly good for inflamed skin conditions and is even reported to be an aphrodisiac. If the result is too heavy, it can be lightened with a few drops of ylang-ylang or citrus oil.

Uses of cosmetic oils include the following:

Shaving oil. When you've found a combination that you like, try using a few drops with lots of warm water to soften the beard rather than using a shaving foam that will remove the natural skin oils. The water and oil mixture is also an excellent moisturiser without the emulsifiers and stabilisers used in commercial moisturisers. When you've finished, use a few drops of the oil as an aftershave. After a few days, you will find that shaving rash is a thing of the past, and you will also find that you will cut yourself less often as the skin begins to strengthen. If shaving rash (or acne) persists, use a little tea tree oil that is a fantastic antimicrobial agent diluted about half and half with a carrier oil.

Deodorants. Stick deodorants are little more than a hard butter containing aroma chemicals. So when you've developed your favourite oil blend, try adding a few drops to a little melted and tempered cocoa or shea butter softened with about 5% olive oil and let it solidify in a stick shape.

Hair. It is somewhat pointless and expensive to use copious quantities of shampoo that remove all the natural hair oil and then use a conditioner to put it all back again. So when you wash your hair, use shampoo very sparingly so as not to remove more of your natural hair oil than necessary, towel the hair to dry it rather than use a hairdryer, and when almost dry, put a couple of drops of Moroccan Argan oil or even your favourite oil blend on your palms and rub it in your scalp before combing the hair. Almond oil is very good also.

Wrinkles. Many ladies spend lots of money on expensive skin preparations that purport to reduce wrinkles. Many of these preparations are based on almond oil and lanolin. Whilst lanolin makes the product smooth and gives it a nice feel; almond oil will generally give just as good results when used every evening. You can buy sweet almond oil from health food shops or pharmacies, but sweet almond is only a variety of the normal almond tree; the oils are very similar, and almond oil can be bought in supermarkets more cheaply.

Nails. Rubbing a little almond oil or your favourite blend onto your nails and into the cuticles, will over time, strengthen them and give a nice sheen without the need for nail varnish.

In short, by doing these things, we are replacing lots of synthetic chemicals in cosmetic preparations with natural oils for nearly all cosmetic applications. Remember, if you can't eat it, you shouldn't be putting it on your skin. And by not removing the natural skin oils with lots of soap, you are less likely to get dry skin and eczema, and wrinkles. Anti-inflammatory foods generally work well from the inside but where the skin is poorly supplied with blood vessels such as on the shins and outer arms, oiling the skin may well reduce or even prevent itching.

Putting It All Together

It's the combination as a whole that works, not odd bits and pieces

In the Introduction, we said there are two nutritional reasons why some people are slim whilst others struggle with their weight:

> **Slim people generally absorb fewer Calories Slim people have faster metabolisms**

We have also seen that it is the high carbohydrate, low fat diets that have been associated with obesity, not high fat, low carbohydrate diets, and many recent studies have confirmed this (18,20,22,). We have also shown that high dietary fat is not the reason for unsightly body fat or coronary heart disease (19,21,23,24,25,26,27,28).

Doing the following, which have all been discussed in previous chapters, will help to achieve both these objectives:

Minimise intake of free sugar including sugar added to manufactured products such as fizzy drinks. Restrict intake of refined carbohydrates such as white bread, cakes, and biscuits.

Consume fruit sparingly and fruit juices hardly at all and eat plenty of lightly cooked vegetables and salads for their antioxidant content. Don't be worried about eating animal fat or full-fat dairy products and choosing butter rather than margarines that are often made with polyunsaturated fats.

Restrict intake of polyunsaturated oils such as sunflower, corn, or safflower oil and use monounsaturated olive or rapeseed oil instead. Eat lots of fresh wild fish, or fish or krill oil. If your blood pressure and blood chemistry are fine, you eat plenty of salads and vegetables, and you don't smoke, don't worry about your blood cholesterol.

Don't worry about salt if you eat lots of vegetables and salads and maximise good HDL cholesterol by doing plenty of exercise. Clean work surfaces with water to remove soil and don't worry about a few bacteria.

Try not to apply things to your skin that you wouldn't eat.

As we said in the chapter on dairy products, milk is a complete food. By analogy, approximately one-third of our food solids should be slowly fermentable carbohydrate and fibre, about one-third fat, and about one-third protein. The traditional dinner of meat or fish, a little potato and lots of vegetables or salad provide exactly that. As in milk, the fat can be saturated fat and monounsaturated oil but aim to keep polyunsaturated oil intake as low as possible. Milk contains nine parts of water to one part of solids, so we should aim to drink plenty of liquid with every meal. Aim also to include several salad and vegetable components with each meal to provide a wide range of minerals and antioxidants. Remember that the vegetable or salad portion of the meal should be as large as the meat or fish and carbohydrate (potatoes, pasta, or grain) portions together.

Remember also that there is no such thing as bad food, only a bad diet, so you may include some naughty things in small amounts as a treat.

So let's conclude with a few suggestions for our main meals.

Suggested breakfasts include:

No added sugar, muesli containing lots of nuts with whole milk

Eggs cooked any way on wholemeal bread or toast spread with butter.

Add tomatoes, mushrooms, and baked beans, if you like. Not too much bacon, other cured meats, or sausage as these may contain nitrites.

Wholemeal bread with cheeses

Porridge with cream

Plenty of tea or coffee without sugar or water

Avoid American breakfasts of waffles and syrups, too much fruit or juice, too much marmalade, jam or honey, and breakfast cereals containing a lot of sugar.

Suggested lunches include:

Soup or broth with cream, if you like it, and wholemeal bread with butter, or sandwich.

Mixed salad with as many components as you can find, such as different sorts of lettuce, tomato, cucumber, olives, radishes, peppers, raw peas, pine nuts, toasted seeds, and raw vegetables, and liberally dressed with olive or rapeseed oil and vinegar or balsamic if you want it. Add meat, fish or egg and wholemeal bread containing nuts and seeds.

Pizza with lots of different components in the topping.

Plenty of tea or coffee without sugar, or water with or without a glass of wine.

Avoid just eating snacks such as cakes, biscuits, and pastries. Have small amounts of these if you've finished your main meal and still feel a bit hungry.

Suggested dinners include:

Meat or fish with potatoes and lots of different vegetables or salads. If you had fish for lunch, choose meat or vice-versa; if you had vegetables for lunch, choose salads or vice-versa.

Curry but with lots of vegetable or salad side dishes

Pasta with lots of tomato and salad

Chinese meal with vegetables such as bamboo shoots, mushrooms, sweet corn, water chestnuts, spring onion, broccoli, beansprouts, or garlic.

Avoid eating processed food too often. Burgers and the like are fine occasionally but not more than once or twice a week.

And if you wish to, enjoy a glass or two of wine, preferably red with your meal. If you drink alcohol, aim preferably for wine mostly with food or just before or just after food. Most of us know that we feel drunk much more quickly when consuming alcohol on an empty stomach. It is absorbed into our system faster than when our stomachs are full during or after eating. It's also the same with food. Grazing, the practice of eating a mouthful or two frequently all during the day, results in far more Calories being absorbed than eating the same amount of food at two or three meal sittings.

So, in summary, we can **avoid unnecessary Calorie absorption by**:

Consuming fats and monounsaturated oils as part of our meal to line our intestines and slow down the absorption of fattening sugars and carbohydrates.

Eating plenty of fibre from vegetables and salads. This promotes a healthy gut microflora, reduces Calorie absorption, and promotes rapid intestinal transit.

Eating conventional meals at breakfast, lunch, and dinner times and avoiding small snacks in between meals and in particular grazing.

We can speed up our metabolisms by:

Getting plenty of exercise, ideally half an hour a day or at least every other day.

Minimising our consumption of sugar and refined (white) carbohydrates.

Not going to bed on a full stomach and getting plenty of sleep.

Not over-eating but consuming fats and oils as part of our meals to keep us feeling replete.

If we were all to follow and stick to these simple rules, I believe that almost anyone can lose weight without food restriction and dieting and, in many cases, prolong their life and its quality. Today some 75% of our food is produced from just twelve plant and five animal species (15). Policy makers and the food industry need to find ways of making it easy for all of us to eat the thirty or more different foodstuffs that some of the more enlightened nutritionists are now saying we need.

A note for vegetarians and vegans

Vegetarians need to be aware that their bodies may become deficient over time in the following that are only found in animal products or to very limited amounts in plant material. You should make special provisions through supplements to make sure you get adequate amounts in your diet.

Vitamin B12, lack of which can cause macrocytic anaemia.

Iron, lack of which can also cause anaemia.

Long chain fish oils (see chapters 7 and 8)

Some amino acids such as carnitine, lysine and methionine.

The mineral zinc and also iodine.

In addition, you may also need vitamin D if you don't get much sunlight.

Vegans may need the following also.

Calcium, lack of which may cause bone or skeletal issues

Choline, found abundantly in eggs, lack of which may cause nerve issues.

Appendix Sports Nutrition

Many books have been written about sports nutrition, so I shall limit myself here to discussing only what the body does when unusual energy demands are made on it and a small amount on protein needs and sources. This is aimed at people doing everyday sports rather than specialist athletes and bodybuilders who will need professional advice.

Energy needs.

The energy needs of active muscles are quite different to those of resting muscle.

In resting muscle, the major fuel source is fat (fatty acids) from adipose tissue that supplies about 85% of the energy requirement.

This is a relatively slow process, so when muscle requires a lot of energy quickly, such as a short sprint, that energy comes initially from glucose taken up from the blood. The heart pumps faster to supply more glucose and also oxygen. This energy process requires a body chemical found in muscle called creatine, commonly sold in health food shops. However, this initial pace can only be sustained for about 5 seconds because the blood creatine level drops about fivefold in this time. Thus the winner of a 10-second sprint is the runner who slows the least. Indeed competitors in events requiring a run-up might consider limiting their approach to around 4 seconds or less to see if their performance improves.

So a second source of energy is required: stored glycogen in leg muscles is broken down to energy, in part without oxygen as this is also a limiting factor. The initial pace must also drop because firstly, the blood lactate level is raised about fivefold, and this causes the familiar ache in muscles that are undergoing heavy exercise. Secondly, this lactic acid makes the blood more acid, which would cause acidosis if the process continued.

So a third source of energy is needed for distance running. The body reverts to fatty acids, which are by far the largest energy source in the body, in fact, over 99% if we ignore protein. Glycogen in muscle accounts for most of the rest, followed by liver glycogen. Initial blood glucose accounts for less than 0.02% hence the 5–6 second limit in a sprint.

The running of distances over about 1km requires cooperation between different energy sources: muscle glycogen, liver glycogen, and fat reserves (adipose tissue). The limiting factor in these events is normally how fast the body can get oxygen to muscles, so lung function and circulation are key. Although the body can extract some energy from glucose and glycogen without oxygen, this is only about 5% of the amount that can be generated with oxygen and the generation rate is slower. There is plenty of energy in adipose tissue even for a marathon, but the generation rate is slower again and at least ten times slower during the initial 5 seconds of a sprint. This means that a marathon would take 5–6 hours to complete if energy came from adipose tissue alone. So the bodies of top athletes consume about equal quantities of adipose tissue and glycogen, the bulk of this aerobically. The use of adipose tissue before too much glycogen is used allows the glycogen store to last until the end of the race. Top sprinters exceed 10 meters per second, whereas top distance runners fall only to about half this speed by using adipose tissue and glycogen most optimally.

Protein requirements.

We have not said much about protein in this book because protein does not significantly contribute to the body's energy balance. Proteins are stored as muscle and are the building blocks of tissue and as such are constantly being recycled. For this purpose, a fist-sized portion of protein per day is an adequate quantity. However, a typical diet provides about twice this amount. For body-building purposes, a fist-sized portion of protein or more should be taken with every meal.

Other things being equal, this protein will go fairly evenly onto all the body muscles. However, suppose you are exercising some muscles more than others, for example, the leg muscles. In that case, if you are a runner, those muscles will show greater development than arm, shoulder, and abdominal muscles.

Good quality protein includes fish, poultry, dairy, lean meat, eggs, and soya. Concentrated protein sources are available as powders, drinks, and bars from health food shops and are mostly made from milk (whey protein) and soya as these are generally the cheapest. Eggs are particularly good and a three-egg omelette made with a variety of vegetable and salad ingredients is particularly good and significantly cheaper than an equivalent weight of steak.

Proteins are composed of amino acids. There are twenty of them in proteins, and many amino acids are essential; that is, we cannot make them in our bodies. Good quality proteins will provide a wide and balanced range of these amino acids. Whilst you can buy specific amino acids in health food shops, it is better not to take these without specialist advice. They can disturb the body's protein balance, and unless you are a specialist bodybuilder, they aren't necessary.

Finally, two warnings. Never take steroids. And remember that alcohol causes fatigue and will impair performance.

References

1. Patel, C quoted by Wilson, C (2019). The only food advice you need. New Scientist 3238, 32-35.
2. Heinonen OP, Albanes D, Virtamo J, et al. Prostate cancer and supplementation with alpha-tocopherol and beta-carotene: incidence and mortality in a controlled trial. J Natl Cancer Inst. 1998;90:440-446.
3. Klein EA, Thompson IM, Jr., Tangen CM, et al. Vitamin E and the risk of prostate cancer: the Selenium and Vitamin E Cancer Prevention Trial (SELECT). JAMA. 2011;306:1549-56.
4. Gaziano J et al. (2009) Vitamins E and C in the prevention of prostate and total cancer in men: the Physicians' Health Study II randomized controlled trial. JAMA. 301, 52-62.
5. Brown D (2005). Unabsorbed calories: an important consideration. Br Med J 330, 7504.
6. De Souza R et al. (2015). Intake of saturated and trans-unsaturated fatty acids and risk of all cause morbidity, cardiovascular disease and type-2 diabetes; systematic review and meta-analysis of observational studies. Br Med J 351, 3978.
7. Chowdhury R et al. (2014). Association of dietary, circulating and supplementary fatty acids with coronary risk; a systematic review and meta-analysis. Ann Intern Med 160, 398-406.
8. Skeaff C and Miller J (2009). Dietary fat and coronary heart disease: summary of evidence from

prospective cohort and randomised controlled trials. Ann Nutr Metab 55, 173-201.

9. Li Y et al. (2015). Saturated fats compared with unsaturated fats and sources of carbohydrates in relation to risk of coronary heart disease: a prospective cohort study. J Am Coll Cardiol 201, 1538-1548.

10. Praagman J et al. (2016). The association between dietary saturated fatty acids and ischaemic heart disease depends on the type and source of fatty acid in the European Prospective Investigation into cancer and nutrition-Netherlands cohort. Am J Clin Nutr 103, 356-365.

11. Anon (2019). Army troops have worse heart health than civilian population. Am Heart Assoc News 5th June, 2019.

12. Gonzalez-Gil E et al. (2017). Ideal vascular health and inflammation in European adolescents: the Helena study. Nutr Metab Card Diseases 27, 447-455.

13. Nakamura Y et al. (2008) Conjugated linoleic acid modulation of risk factors associated with atherosclerosis. Nutr Metab 5, 22.

14. Ochoa J et al. (2004). Conjugated linoleic acids (CLAs) decrease prostrate cancer cell proliferation. Carcinogenesis 25, 1185-1191.

15. Fernandez M. (2012). Rethinking dietary cholesterol. Curr Opin Clin Nutr Metab Care 15, 117-121.

16. Goodwin J (2021). How to keep your brain blooming. New Scientist 250 (3330), 38-42.

17. Simopoulos A. (2002). The importance of the ratio of omega-6/omega-3 essential fatty acids. Biomed Pharmacother. 56, 365-379.

18. Hession M et al. (2009). Systematic review of randomised controlled trials of low carbohydrate

vs.low-fat/low-calorie diets in the management of obesity and its comorbilities. Obes Rev. 10, 36-50.

19. Siri-Tarino P et al. (2015). Saturated fats versus carbohydrates for cardiovascular disease prevention. Ann Rev Nutr 17, 517-543.

20. Forsythe C et al. (2010). Limited effect of dietary saturated fat on plasma saturated fat in the context of a low carbohydrate diet. Lipids 45, 947-962

21. Siri-Tarino P et al. (2010). Saturated fat, carbohydrate and cardiovascular disease. Am J Clin Nutr 91, 502-509.

22. Willett WC (2002). Dietary fat is not a major determinant of body fat. Am. J Med. 13, 47-59.

23. Chowdhury R et al. (2014). Association of dietary, circulating and supplementary fatty acids with coronary risk: a systematic review and meta-analysis. Ann Intern Med. 160, 398-406.

24. Menotti A et al. (1999). Food intake patterns and 25-year mortality from coronary heart disease: cross-cultural correlations in the Seven Countries Study. Eur J Epidemiol. 15, 507-515.

25. Santos F et al. (2012). Systematic review and meta-analysis of clinical trials of the effects of low carbohydrate diets on cardiovascular risk factors. Obes Rev. 13, 1048-1066.

26. Leaf A. (1999). Dietary prevention of coronary heart disease: the Lyon Diet Heart Study. Circulation 16, 733-735.

27. Kris-Etherton P etal (2001). American Heart Association science advisory: Lyon Diet Heart Study. Circulation 103, 1823-1825.

28. Oh K et al. (2005). Dietary fat intake and risk of coronary heart disease in women: 20 years of follow-up of the nurses' health study. Am J Epidemiology 161, 672-679.